CONTENTS

GABRIELE BURACCHI

DETOX DIET IN THE ZONE

Purify and detoxify yourself using nutrition

Dr. Gabriele Buracchi
Nutrizionista e Psicologo

DETOX

After many decades that I have known and applied the Zone diet, this diet and lifestyle continues to fascinate me for its many applications and variations.

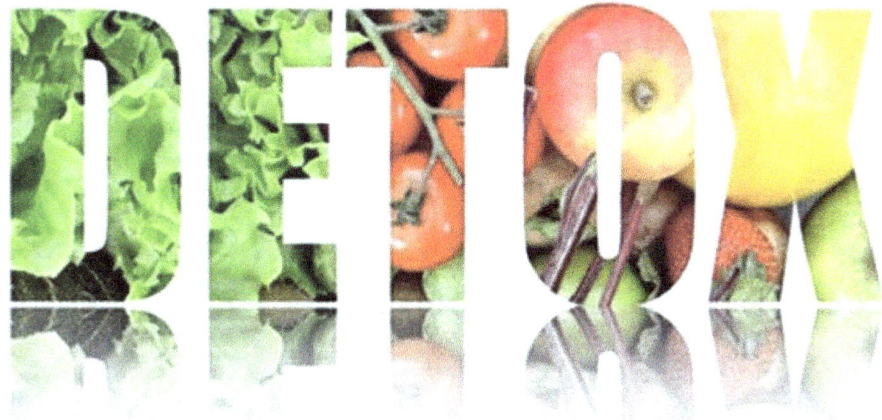

One of these applications is the Detox diet, or the application of the principles of the Zone to this diet, its relationships between Carbohydrates, Proteins and Fats but also the necessary physical activity and relaxation. Let's start by trying to understand what it is for: It is used to detoxify the body when, for various reasons, our diet has been unbalanced, rich in saturated or trans fats and foods that acidify our body, producing a condition of acidity and toxicity due to the accumulation of waste in the body.

And let us see also to those who need it:

It is used by all those people who often find themselves eating in an unregulated way, without paying attention to the quality of the food or, even, when it happens to have a wrong diet even on the weekend alone to purify the body and start eating well in the Zone again.

So let's begin to see first the Detox and then the Zone in order to be able to put them together in a productive way.

Detox Diet in the Zone.

An important resource for eliminating waste and toxins from the body while remaining in the Zone.

A question can arise spontaneously.

But Why Should I Do A Detox Diet?

Unfortunately, it is a fairly generalized observation that the hectic life that most of us lead, with the consequent lack of time to buy and cook natural products, leads more and more often to consume foods that are quick to prepare, but preserved, unfortunately rich in known and less known additives.

Maybe this can happen even if the quantitative parameters 40/30/30 of the Zone are respected but not the qualitative ones.

Just to give a simple example, the **Zone diet** tells me that, for example, for a main meal, I have 3 blocks, so I have to choose my three C mini blocks or Carbohydrate Blocks.

If formally, from the point of view of the Zone tables these three mini-blocks could indifferently consist of 900 g. of Asparagus or just 30g. of Wafer, it is clear that even if formally it is the same thing, in practice they will be two very different choices.

In the second case it is a qualitatively unbalanced choice, rich in saturated fats, dyes and preservatives, certainly able to acidify our body, producing a condition of acidity and toxicity due to the accumulation of waste in the tissues. And, from another point o view,) 900g of Asparagus can full the belly, while 30g. of wafer will leave you hungry.

In particular, two fundamental systems for well-being are involved:

1) the digestive system, with various problems of digestion, reflux, intestinal slowdown and constipation up to inflammatory diseases

2) the circulatory system which, particularly in women, is suffering with signs of lymphoedema and heaviness

as well as obvious imperfections such as swelling of the ankles and cellulite.

It happens on numerous occasions for lunches or dinners with friends, parties, weddings, children's birthdays and Saturday night pizza.

It is not possible to give up all this, and certain occasions *can and must* continue to exist, because they are moments of leisure and sociality and it is right to enjoy them.

Precisely for this reason, if serious allergies or intolerances that require a specific dietary regime are not diagnosed, even on the occasions mentioned above, it is useful to carry out a Detox or Detoxifying diet cycle after each period of food "*distractions*".

The Detox or Detox diet, thanks to the elimination of waste accumulated in the tissues, helps to be more deflated, to regain a sense of lightness that manifests itself in a better physical and mental shape.

Of course Detox, but in the Zone

If certain errors occur frequently, you can also get into the habit of following the Detox Zone diet for 2 days a week, such as:

Monday and Tuesday as a weekend recovery.

The Detox Zone diet thus becomes a tool for preventing

chronic and inflammatory diseases, thus allowing to slow down the aging process which, on the contrary, is favored by a diet rich in sugars and saturated fats.

Furthermore, thanks to the absence of refined sugars and saturated fats as well as the reduced caloric intake and the use of highly digestible proteins, the Detox Zone diet facilitates weight loss from the very first days.

It is also a help in those who suffer from severe water retention.

Many demonize proteins and perhaps some think that a detox diet should be free of it.

Nothing more false.

Proteins are the basic constituent of our body - except water,we are mainly made of proteins - what matters is the quality of the proteins we ingest.

The Detox Zone Diet provides proteins mainly from fish and uses plant-based proteins such as soy, bamboo, almonds, legumes etc.

It can also be safely followed by vegetarians and vegans.

The Detox Zone diet, due to its structure, lends itself to last for periods of one or two weeks, to then be replaced with a Mediterranean Zone diet, also a variant of the very favorable Zone.

As already mentioned, it can also be simply used for a couple of days a week, in this case for indefinite periods.

Foods to avoid: cold cuts, cheeses, red meats, fried, white bread and bread, pasta, rice, sugar, sweets especially after dinner, alcohol.

Foods to be preferred: fish of all kinds, especially blue fish. Proteins of vegetable origin from Soy, Lupins, Bamboo, Almonds, Legumes. Use only very occasionally: white meats, low-fat cheeses (primo sale, ricotta, goat).

Some of these foods are discussed in the second part of the book. If necessary to sweeten, use STEVIA, even if getting used to the true tastes of foods without additions still involves an increase in awareness.

Do not forget 2 liters of water a day and at least 45 minutes of physical activity daily to expel toxins.

These are the general concepts. Let's now look at some practical applications needed to undertake the detoxification process.

DETOXIFYING HERBAL TEA

To purify yourself to the best

In addition to the Zone Detox Diet, there are some other things we can do to detoxify the body to an even greater extent.

One of these are Detox Teas.

Here I provide some general indications of the active ingredients that I consider most useful.

Surely your herbalist will be able to advise you best.

These Detox Teas can be used during the period of a couple of weeks of the diet, but they can become a good daily habit, to be maintained.

So let's review the main herbs used to prepare detoxifying herbal teas.

It is also good to point out that herbal teas should not be counted in the diet.

They are a great ally of the liver because they help in the purifying action.

They also have an interesting effect on hypercholesterolemia.

ARTICHOKE (Cynara scolymus).

The infusion or herbal tea prepared with **artichoke leaves** have important properties from the point of view of stimulating diuresis and eliminating toxins.

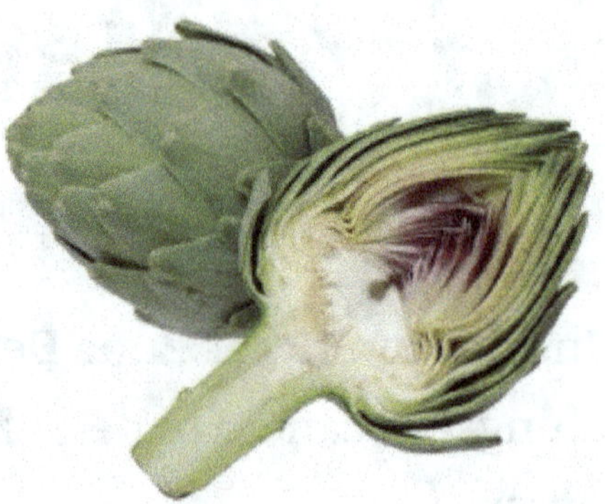

The taste is very bitter, but the benefit is assured, as the belly deflates, excess fluids are eliminated, circulation is reactivated.

Artichoke contains **Cynarin**, an active ingredient that promotes diuresis and biliary secretion, allowing the liver to be purified.

It is the purifying herb par excellence, one of the best detoxifying herbal teas.

There are two parts that we can use: the leaf and the root, and both to regulate the digestive system.

We can prepare an infusion of leaves, or make an herbal tea with toasted roots, more useful for liver problems.

Both experimental and clinical effects have been verified through extensive research on biomedical herbal remedies.

In particular, antioxidant, choleretic, hepatoprotective, biliary and lipid-lowering effects have been demonstrated, which corresponded to its historical use.

Ongoing research seems to indicate that the artichoke does indeed have medicinal qualities.

The most significant appears to be its beneficial effect on the liver.

Purifying herbal tea with artichoke:

40 gr of artichoke, stem or root, infused in hot water.

Strain and drink, up to three cups a day, before meals.

Bibliography.

Pharmacological Studies of Artichoke Leaf Extract and Their Health Benefits

https://link.springer.com/article/10.1007/s11130-015-0503-8

DANDELION (Taraxacum officinale).

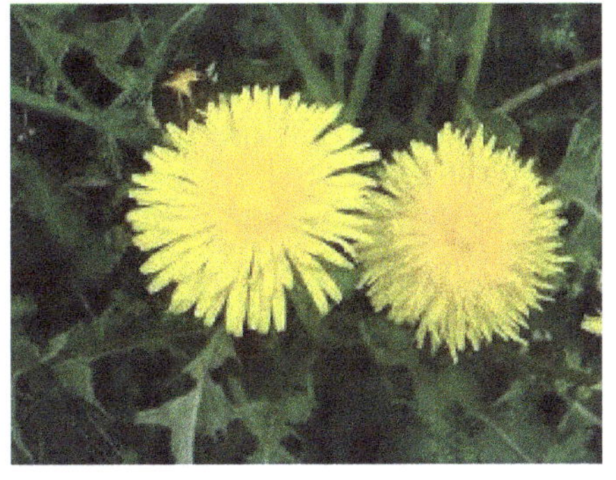

It is the purifying herb par excellence, one of the best detoxifying herbal teas.

There are two parts that we can use: the leaf and the root, both of which regulate the digestive system.

We can prepare an infusion of leaves, or make an herbal tea with toasted roots, more useful for liver problems.

Dandelion has diuretic properties and improves digestion.

Roots and **leaves** are very rich in potassium which promotes drainage and elimination of excess fluids, counteracting water retention and thus purifying the urinary tract.

Detoxifies and cleanses the liver.

The therapeutic effects most often found in the scientific literature are antioxidant, hepatoprotective and antitumor effects.

Dandelion purifying herbal tea:

25 grams of dried leaves in a jug of water.

Leave to infuse for 6 minutes, covered, filter and drink.

Minimum two cups a day.

Alternatively: 50 gr. of leaves for a liter of water to drink throughout the day.

Bibliography.

A comprehensive review of the benefits of Taraxacum officinale on human health https://bnrc.springeropen.com/articles/10.1186/s42269-021-00567-1

BIRCH (Betula alba)

It is an excellent blood purifier, it frees the body from toxins, stagnation of liquids and excess uric acid.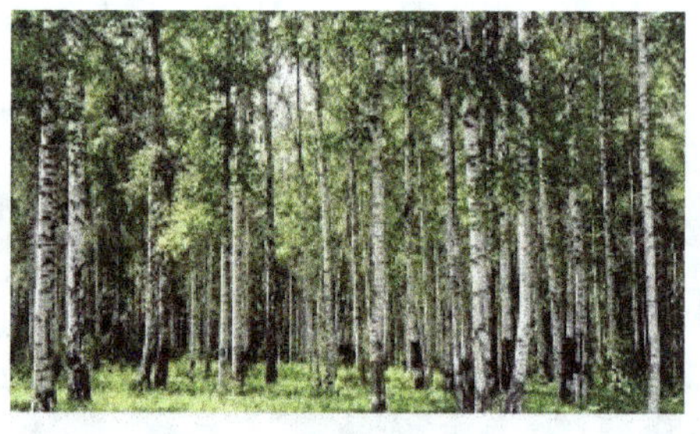
The leaves and buds are rich in flavonoids, essential oil, tannins, sesquiterpene oxides, vitamin C, saponins and much more.

The bark, on the other hand, has a high presence of

triterpenes, betulin and tannins.

Given these concentrations, birch is a natural remedy useful for purification and diuresis, but also as a first-line find for its anti-inflammatory and antiseptic action.

Multiple studies have shown that Birch has various pharmacological activities such as antimalarial, antitumor, antimicrobial and anti-inflammatory.

Birch detox tea: 30 grams of dried and chopped leaves in a jug of water, leave to infuse for five minutes, filter and drink.

Up to three cups a day.

Bibliography.

Phytochemical Constituents and Pharmacological Activities of Betula alba Linn.- A Review

https://www.researchgate.net/profile/Mukesh-Singh-8/
publication/265942129_Phytochemical_Constituents_and_Pharmacological_
Activities_of_Betula_alba_Link1-Activities_of_Betula_alba_Link1-
Activities_of_Betula_alba_Link1-
Activities_of_Betula_alba_Link120fharmological-   Activities-of-Betula-alba-
Linn-A-Review.pdf

NETTLE (Urtica dioica).

It is another herb with great purifying potential, it is also rich in mineral salts and folic acid.

It is a possible natural remedy for the prostate,

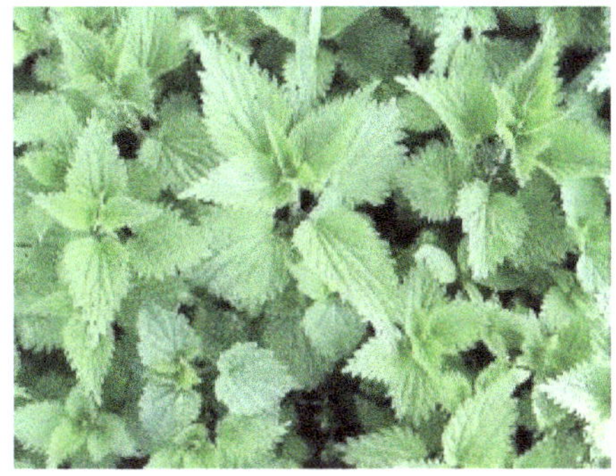

especially in cases of swelling of the prostate gland and pain associated with difficulty in urinating.

Also useful against cystitis. The iron and vitamin C content makes it also recommended for anemia.

It also has vasoconstrictive properties, useful in hypothetical subjects, to which it adds effective healing qualities in the treatment of gastric ulcers and nasal epistaxis (loss of nosebleed) and hemorrhoids with blood loss.

Its leaves are rich in fiber, minerals, vitamins and antioxidant compounds such as polyphenols and carotenoids, as well as antioxidant compounds such as polyphenols and carotenoids.

Nettle has antiproliferative, anti-inflammatory, antioxidant, analgesic, anti-infectious, hypotensive and anti-ulcer characteristics, as well as the ability to prevent cardiovascular disease, in all parts of the plant (leaves, stems, roots and seeds).

Purifying herbal tea with nettle:

25 grams of dried nettle leaves. Leave to infuse for five minutes and drink.

One cup a day after meals.

Bibliography

Nutritional and pharmacological importance of stinging nettle (Urtica dioica L.): A review

https://www.sciencedirect.com/science/article/pii/S2405844022010052

In addition to these individual herbal teas we can also make compotes, to amplify the therapeutic and detoxifying effects.

2 Detox herbal teas mix to purify

1) mix of herbs in herbal tea cut, consisting of: 30 g of pilosella, 20 g of fumitory, 20 g of milk thistle, 20 g of dandelion, 10 g of mint.
Bring 1 heaping tablespoon per cup of water to a boil and leave to infuse for 10 minutes.
Drink 2-3 cups a day.

2) mix of herbs in herbal tea cut: 30 g of horsetail, 30 g of nettle, 20 g of burdock, 20 g of fumitory.

Use one tablespoon per cup of boiling water of this mix. Leave it to infuse for 5-10 minutes, filter and drink. The ideal time is in the morning on an empty stomach. To be taken in the 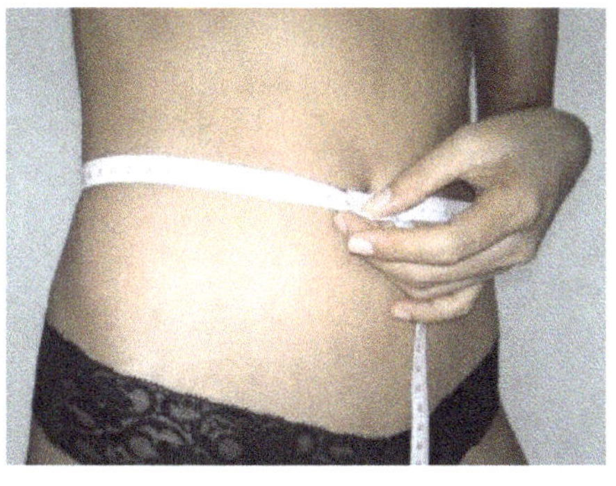 recommended doses and under medical supervision only in case you suffer from particular pathologies.

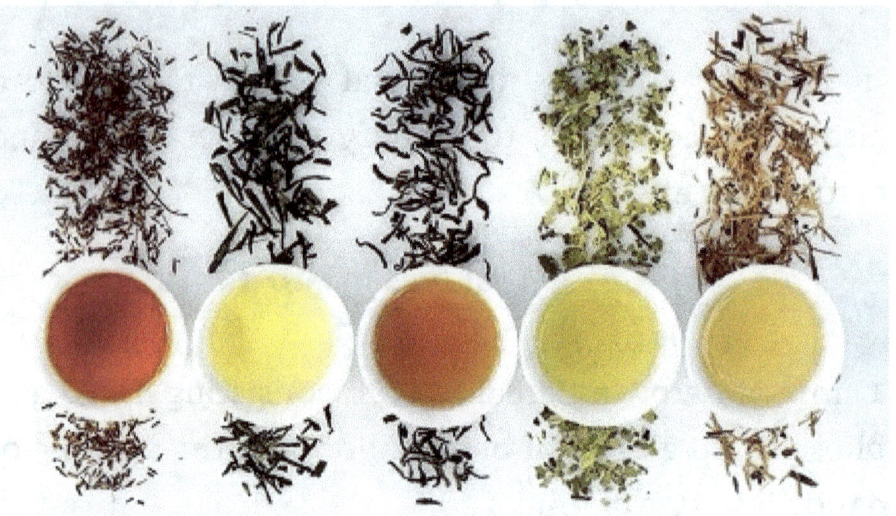

DETOX CENTRIFUGATES

*Purify yourself with fruit
and vegetables*

Detox Centrifugates are natural drinks that are very useful for purifying the body and helping to lose weight because they allow you to get rid of toxins as well as provide valuable vitamins and minerals.

Better to use cold juice extractors that keep many micronutrients such as vitamins and antioxidants that are normally lost with the high revolutions of the blender or traditional centrifuges.

They make vitamins immediately available to our body without straining the digestive system and are certainly better than packaged fruit juices and other sugary drinks found in the supermarket.

Those who want to start a Detox diet in the Zone, perhaps even to lose weight, can use centrifuged as beneficial drinks that can enrich the body with precious substances.

Recipes of centrifuged to prepare at home.

A) Celery and Carrots.

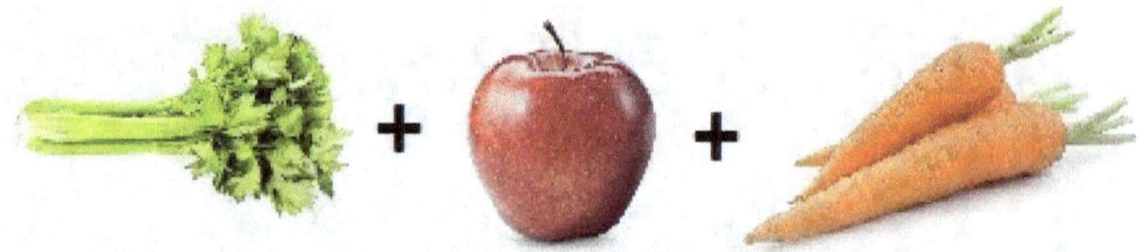

With 3 celery stalks, 1 apple, 1 sprig of parsley, 4 spinach leaves, 1 carrot Cucumbers and celery are among the most useful ingredients for making centrifuged drinks to purify the body.

If you want you can replace the apple with the pear, according to the fruit at your disposal and according to your tastes.

B) Tomato and Apple.

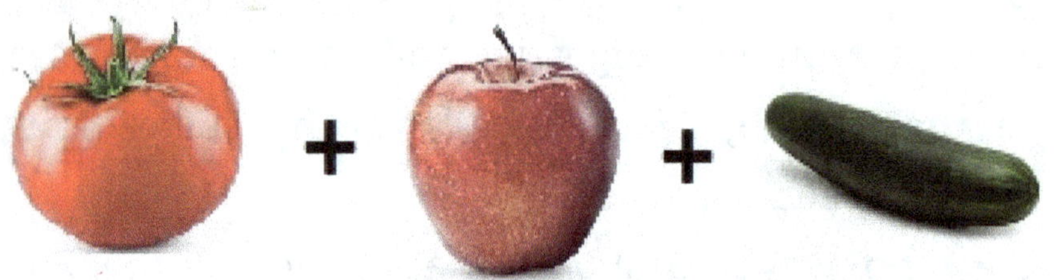

With 1 tomato, 1 apple, 1 cucumber.

It is particularly suitable for summer, due to the seasonality of its ingredients and is useful for its detoxifying action.

C) Parsley and Carrots.

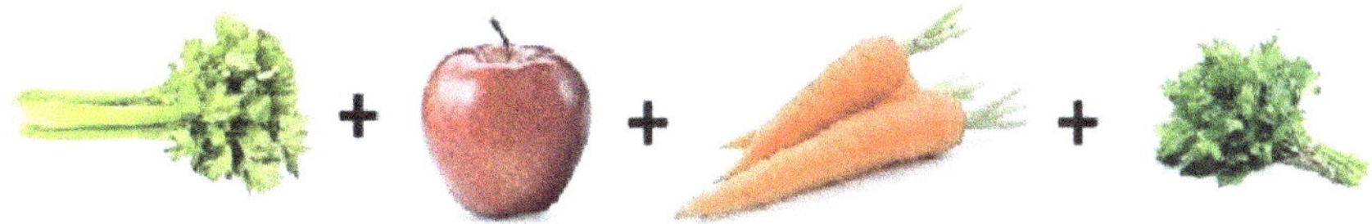

With 1 nice bunch of fresh parsley, 2 carrots, 1 apple, 1 celery stalk.

The parsley used together with the other ingredients helps the body recover energy and get rid of accumulated toxins.

The chlorophyll in parsley helps re-oxygenate the blood. This juice is rich in vitamin C, iron, potassium and calcium.

D) Oranges and Kiwis.

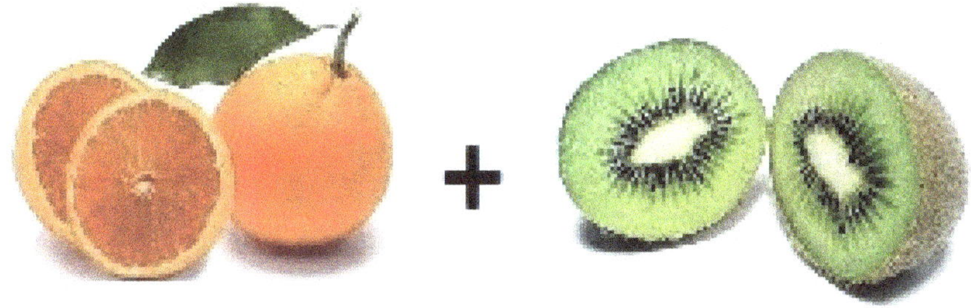

With 2 oranges, 3 kiwis. Both fruits are rich in vitamin C. This juice will help the body to stock up on potassium and vitamin K.

It is a juice that is useful for reducing cholesterol, for increasing iron absorption and for purifying the body.

E) Carrot and Apple.

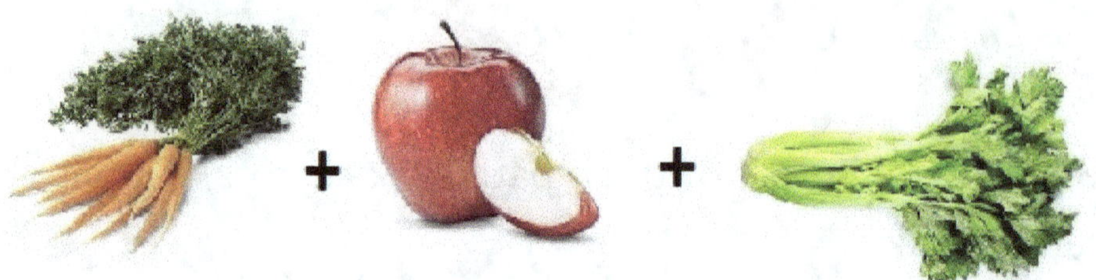

With 2 carrots, 1 apple, 1 celery stalk. It allows you to combine the beneficial properties of apples and carrots, both rich in vitamins, with the detoxifying action of celery.

In addition to the celery stalk, you can also add a few of its leaves.

F) Apple, Pear and Lemon.

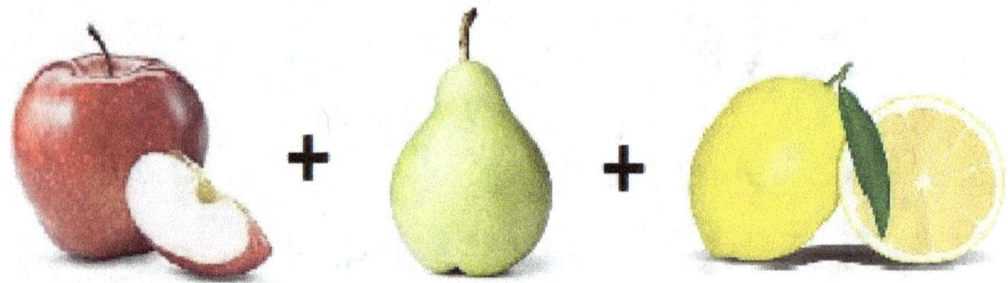

With 1 lemon, 2 apples, 2 pears. Take advantage of the purifying properties of lemon and its juice. Lemon juice has a rather sour taste which is compensated for by combining it with ripe apples and pears.

G) Spinach, Celery, Cucumber, Apple.

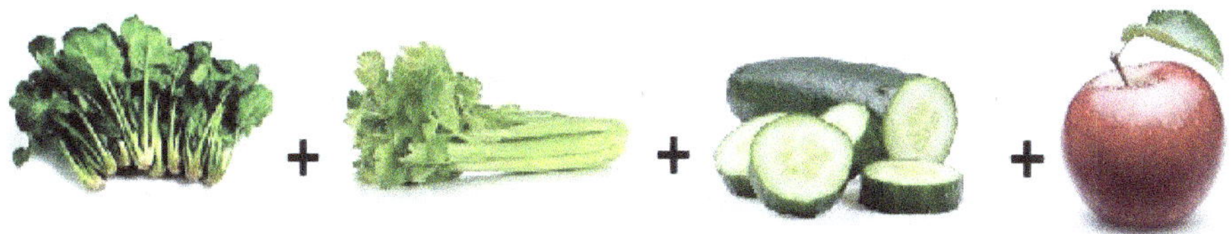

With 50 g of spinach, a stalk of celery, a small cucumber, 2 apples. Centrifuged with a nice bright green color, great for getting back into shape.

Don't add sugar.

Even if it is carbohydrates, the intake of a centrifuged is so low that it may very well not be counted.

DETOX WATER

To cleanse the body

Detox water is a drink that has been known for several years now, also thanks to the success of the Detox diet, from whose principles it derives.

n the collective imagination, water has always been considered as something that cleans, purifies, and marketing has often taken possession of it. 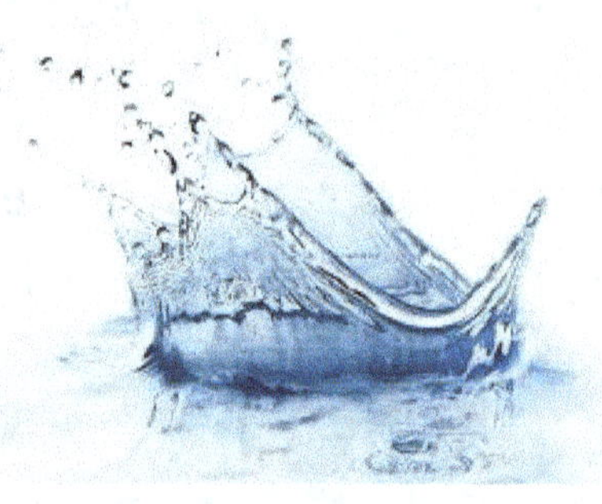
But despite all these properties of water are real.

When the need arises to "get back in place" and detoxify, perhaps from some extravagance such as the use of caloric foods, rich in fats and salt, a few glasses too much, drugs, allergies and intolerances that can burden the body or, maybe, after a period of stress, it may be time to detoxify.

The body, in fact, in the presence of waste and toxins uses the retention of liquids as a defense weapon to "dilute" them and try to make them more "harmless", thus transporting them to the excretory organs (skin, lungs, liver, kidneys , the lymphatic system, etc.) to allow its elimination. Water has many beneficial effects on our body:

fights retention
facilitates the work of the kidneys
eliminates toxins
helps digestion
reduces swelling
reduces nervous hunger
promotes a sense of satiety
stimulates the metabolism to use fat faster

We should drink about two liters a day, but not everyone is capable of it and for this reason I thought it best to combine the properties of water with those of fruit, vegetables, aromatic herbs and spices, creating **Detox Water**.

Of course, we must also combine water with a detox diet in the area to maximize the effects.

How to prepare Detox Water?

Basically it is a question of taking a jug pouring 2 liters of mineral water and adding thinly sliced fruit and vegetables, spices, aromas, leaving everything to rest covered for one night in the fridge.

The next day it will be enough to filter and transfer everything in a bottle for greater convenience.

During the night, at least part of the vitamins and mineral salts will pass from the vegetables to the water, making it rich in beneficial properties as well as giving it taste and aroma without the need to add sugars and calories.

On the appropriate page you can find 5 recipes, although it is still possible to indulge yourself by following your own tastes.

For the avoidance of doubt, it is good to clarify that these are not magical potions and that they cannot even be seen as the solution to long periods of extravagance, but they are certainly an aid to drink more, increase diuresis and eliminate excess retention.

Finally, let us remember that vitamins are labile, so it is best to drink Detox Water as soon as possible.

Detox water is not counted in the diet

Detox Water Recipes.

5 simple recipes to deflate the belly and detoxify, but not only, being rich in vitamins, salts, antioxidants, easy to make and good to drink and useful complement to the diet.

N.B. It is recommended, for all recipes, to start with

organic farming products.

A) Detox Water with Apple and Cinnamon.

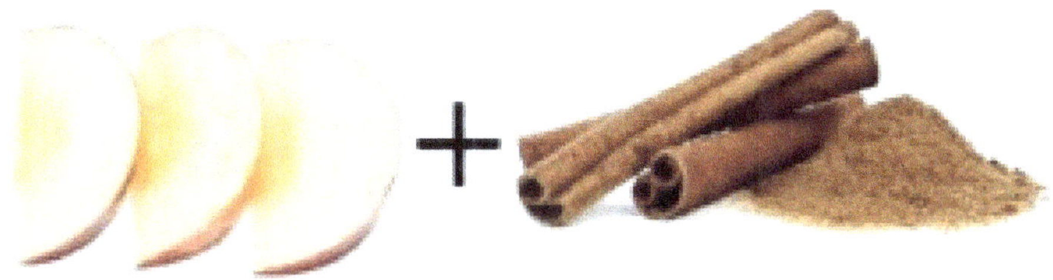

Put 2 apples cut into thin slices with the peel in a jug with 2 liters of water.

Add 2 cinnamon sticks or a couple of teaspoons of ground cinnamon, as this spice has a regulating effect on blood sugar and fight nervous hunger.

Apples are rich in vitamin C and B vitamins and potassium which regulates blood pressure. It is left to rest, shaking every now and then, all night.

B) Detox Water with Cucumber, Lemon and Mint

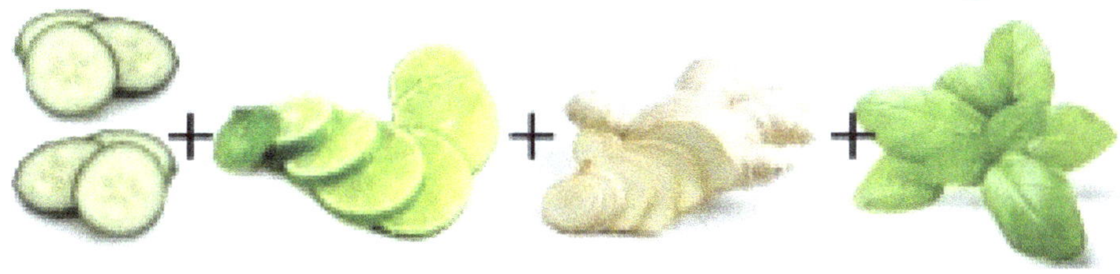

In a jug with 2 liters of water, dip 1 organic lemon cut into slices with all the peel and 10-12 well washed fresh mint leaves as well as 1 medium cucumber cut into slices.

Cucumber is very purifying and detoxifying, but it also contains tartaric acid, an aid in not transforming excess carbohydrates into fat.

Lemon is rich in vitamin C, a powerful antioxidant and citric acid, which helps the liver detoxify, aids digestion, dissolves gallstones, calcium deposits from the kidneys and helps purify the skin.

Mint, thanks to menthol, helps digestion and is useful in case of gastro-intestinal swelling and in reducing irritable bowel spasms. It is left to rest, shaking every now and then, all night.

C) Detox Water with Strawberries and Mint.

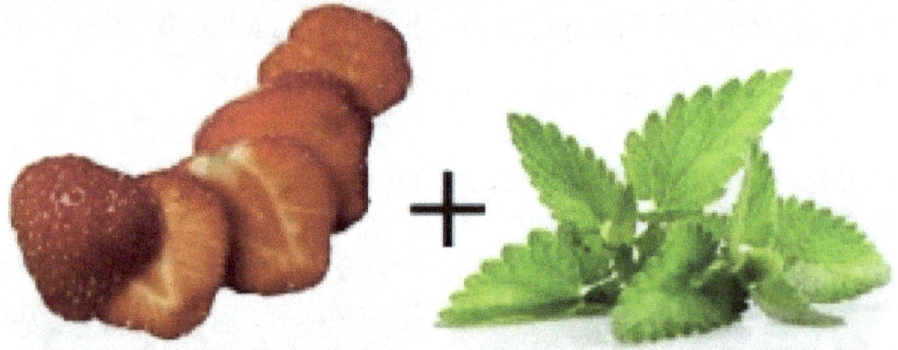

Put 5 sliced strawberries with 6 fresh mint leaves and, preferably, a few slices of lemon in a jug with 2 liters of water.

Strawberries are very rich in antioxidants and in particular in vitamin C, like lemon which also promotes digestion, while mint acts as a carminative against abdominal swelling.

It is left to rest, shaking every now and then, all night.

D) Detox Water with Green Tea, Mint and Lime.

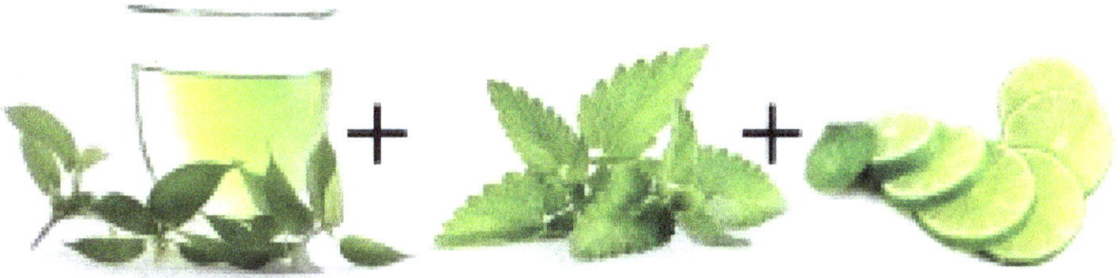

First, a green tea must be prepared by infusing 20 g of leaves in 2 liters of water at 70 ° for 3-4 minutes.

It is important that the water does not boil or the green tea will lose its properties and become bitter.

Green tea is very rich in antioxidants and in particular in epigallocatechin gallate (EGCG), a very powerful antioxidant.

EGCG helps regulate LDL cholesterol levels in the blood.

Lime is very rich in vitamin C, tartaric acid, B vitamins, potassium and magnesium.

Thanks to the potassium, lime is deflating, purifying and energizing. Green tea, mint and lime can be the Detox water suitable for those who are following a diet and want to both drain and lose weight, as well as deflate the belly and detoxify.

Let it all cool down and then put it in the fridge for one

night.

E) Detox Water with Cucumber, Lime, Ginger and Basil.

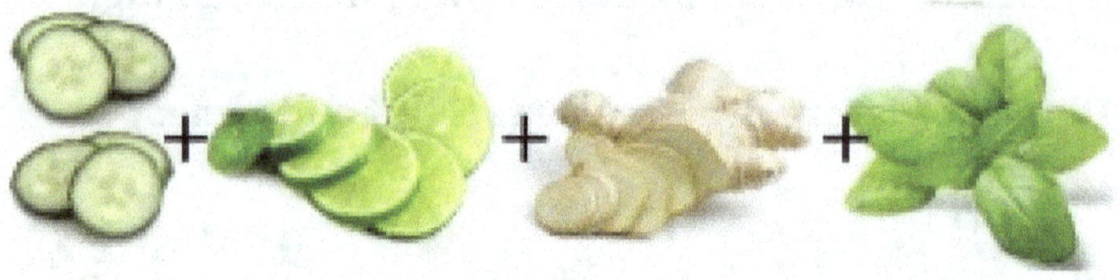

Put the thin slices of 2 limes in a jug with 2 liters of water, 1small cucumber, 10 slices of ginger and 10 large basil leaves.

In addition to deflate the belly and detoxify, Lime contains vitamins especially C and B6, flavonoids, folic acid and potassium with high anti-inflammatory and antioxidant power; reduces blood cholesterol levels; helps digestion and regulates intestinal activity; ideal as a slimming aid.

The peel of the cucumber is very rich in minerals (especially iron, potassium, magnesium and phosphorus) and vitamins (C, A, and group B); if taken regularly it is a valid ally in problems related to hypertension and is diuretic and purifying the liver.

Ginger is digestive, very useful in preventing the formation of abdominal gas and effective against cold symptoms (sore throat and cold).

It also strengthens the immune system and has antipain properties, providing relief in cases of migraine and menstrual pain.

It also has antibiotic properties.

Basil is rich in beta-carotene, so it protects the skin from the harmful effects of the sun and is useful for the health of the cardiovascular system.

It increases the health of skin and hair and helps in case of flatulence and abdominal cramps. It is also a powerful natural antibacterial.

Detox water is not included in the block count of the Detox Zone diet.

EAT THE 5 COLORS

Antioxidants.

If you want to fill up on Antioxidants, absolutely precious and indispensable elements for our health and to detoxify in a profound way, I have prepared many useful indications, especially those useful for consuming fruit and vegetables of the 5 colors, that is that set of foods that allow you to have all types of Antioxidants available, without having any deficiencies. For each color you will also find explained what are the possible benefits for your health, benefits that are well known on the basis of rigorous scientific studies.

What are the benefits.

Eating 5 daily servings of fresh fruit and vegetables in 5 different colors helps keep fit and reduces the risk of developing some serious diseases by a third.

But eating 5 portions of fruit and vegetables also puts us in a position to receive the necessary mini-blocks of carbohydrates from excellent foods and not from bread, pasta and various sugars.

Why the 5 colors?

Because the colors of the diet represent an important source of well-being for our health, contributing to the proper functioning of the human body. The various colors actually represent different types of Antioxidants.

Red.

Red fruits and vegetables are distinguished, first of all, by their important antioxidant properties and their ability to prevent cancer and cardiovascular diseases, also protecting the epithelial tissue.

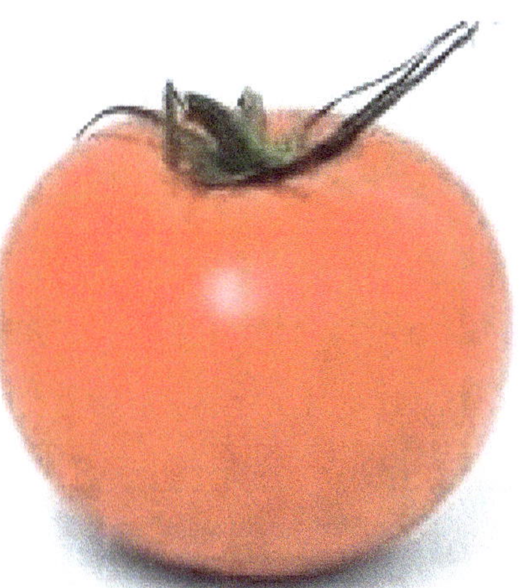

Tomato and its derivatives are the major dietary source of Lycopene.

Here Lycopene represents up to 60% of the total Carotenoid content.

The lycopene content is influenced by the level of ripeness. In red and ripe tomatoes there are 50 mg / kg of Lycopene, a concentration that drops to 5 mg / kg in the yellow varieties.

Other natural sources of Lycopene are melons, guava and pink grapefruits.

The concentration of lycopene in human serum depends on the prolonged intake of these foods.

The bioavailability of the compound appears to be

higher in heat-treated products like tomato sauces versus raw products.

Lycopene, like other carotenoids, has cancer prevention activities.

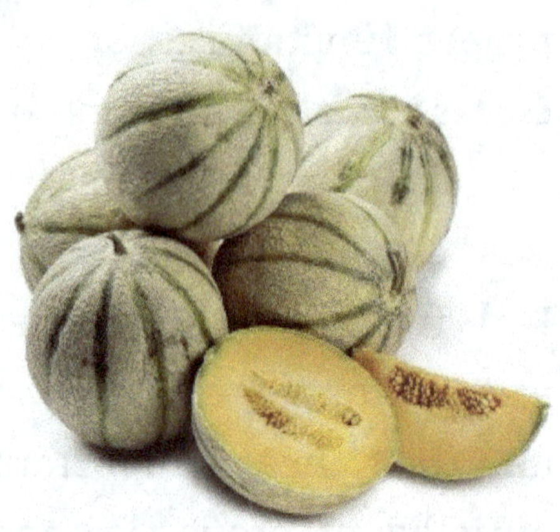

Several studies attribute to Lycopene the ability to reduce the risk of prostate cancer in humans, and the ability to suppress the growth of breast cancer cells.

Lycopene, contained mainly in tomatoes and watermelon, fights breast and ovarian cancers in women and prostate cancer in men.

Anthocyanins and **Carotenoids**, of which blood oranges, strawberries and cherries are particularly rich, are an excellent adjuvant in the treatment of

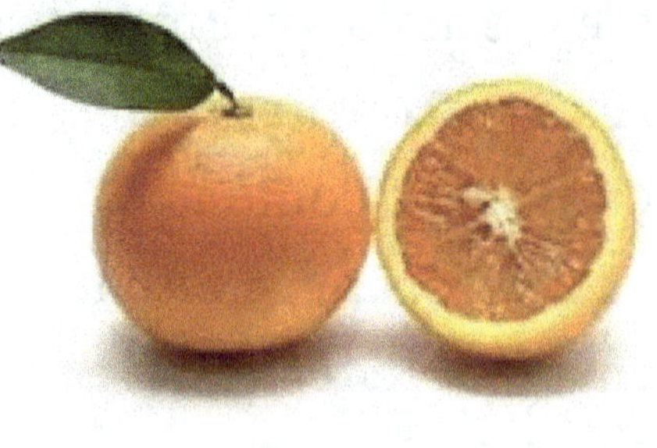

blood vessel diseases and / or capillary fragility, prevent atherosclerosis due to high cholesterol levels and enhance vision.

Furthermore, red foods are the richest in Vitamin C: they promote the production of collagen,

keep blood vessels intact, stimulate the immune system

and wound healing.

Vitamin C is also one of the main responsible for the good absorption of the iron contained in fruit and vegetables.

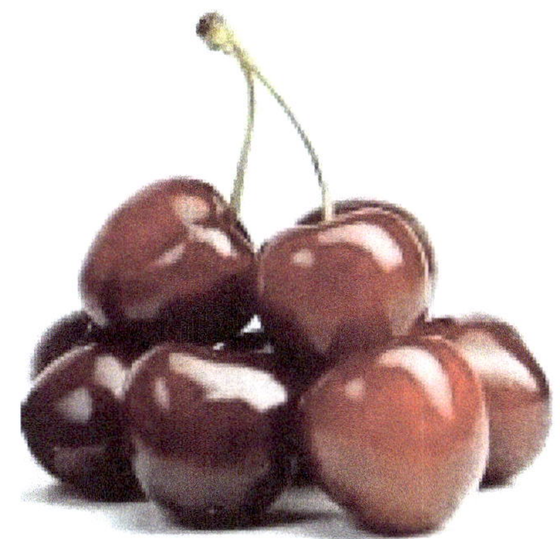

Yellow-orange.

Like red foods, yellow-orange fruits and vegetables help prevent cancer, cardiovascular diseases and cellular aging, also enhancing vision.

Flavonoids are the secret of these effects.

These substances, in fact, act mainly at the gastrointestinal level,

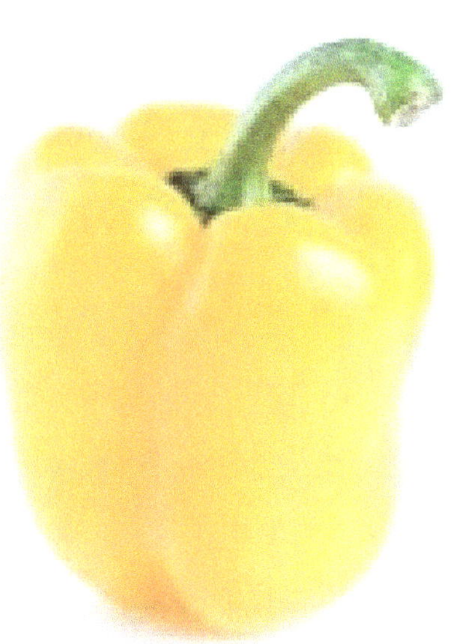

neutralizing the formation of free radicals.

The high content of beta-carotene also protects the body from damage due to the presence of free radicals: moreover, it is absorbed with fats without the risk of overdose, as can happen through excessive use of dietary supplements.

Betacarotene also has a powerful provitamin and antioxidant action and is a precursor of **Vitamin A**, which is important for growth, reproduction, 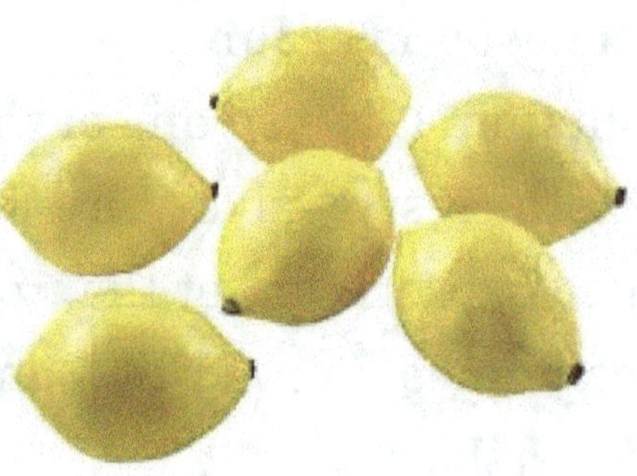 tissue maintenance and immune functions. Peppers, lemons and oranges are particularly rich in **Vitamin C** and have a high antioxidant function and contribute to the production of collagen.

Finally, the anthocyanins contained in these foods (especially oranges) have an anti-inflammatory, antitumor and anticoagulant action.

Green.

Chlorophyll, responsible for the green color of fruit and vegetables, has a powerful antioxidant action, while the carotenoids contained in these foods help the body defend itself and prevent coronary heart disease and many types of cancer; in addition, they are responsible for the sight and development of epithelial cells.

These foods are particularly rich in Magnesium, a very important mineral: it promotes the metabolism of carbohydrates and proteins, stimulates the absorption of Calcium, Phosphorus, Sodium and Potassium, regulates blood vessel pressure and the transmission of nervous impulse.

Green leafy vegetables are a great source of folic acid (and folate), useful as a preventive tool against atherosclerosis and, in the case of new

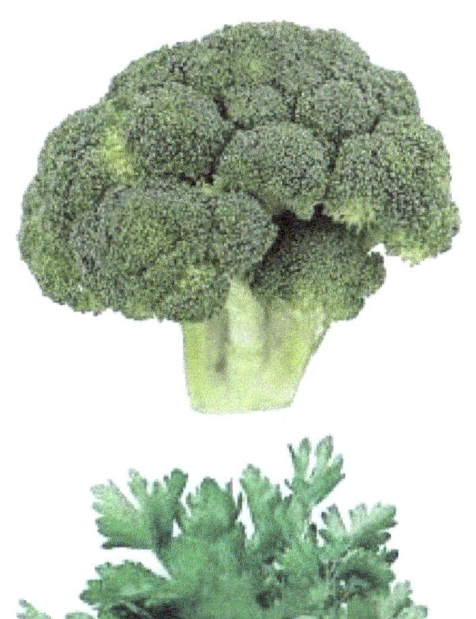

borns, the risk of incomplete closure of the vertebral canal during pregnancy.

Broccoli, parsley, spinach and kiwi are very rich in Vitamin C: they therefore favor the absorption of the iron contained in fruit and vegetables, and have

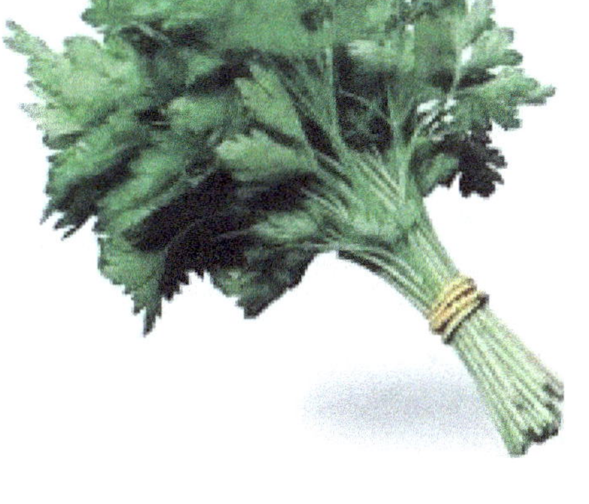

antioxidant properties and help prevent cardiovascular, neurological and cancer diseases.

Blue-violet.

lue-violet foods, in addition to protecting eyesight (especially blueberries) and preventing tumors and cardiovascular diseases, contribute to a correct urinary function (especially berries). An important antioxidant action is carried out by anthocyanins, which defend the body from pathologies due to poor blood circulation, protecting the capillaries.

They prevent atherosclerosis caused by high cholesterol levels and inhibit platelet aggregation.

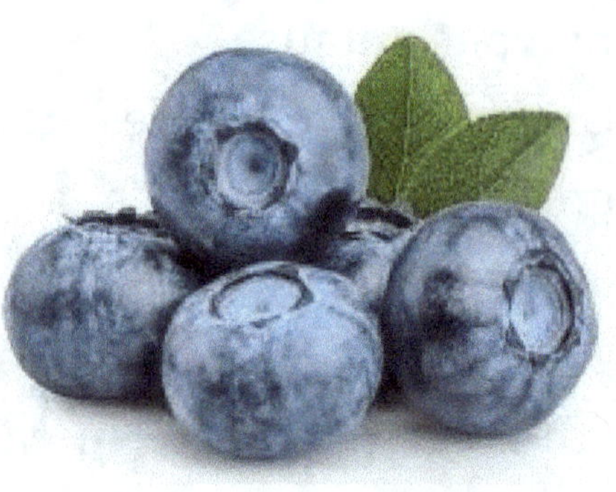

Currants and radicchio, in addition to the antioxidant properties due to the presence of Vitamin C, intervene in the formation of carnitine and collagen.

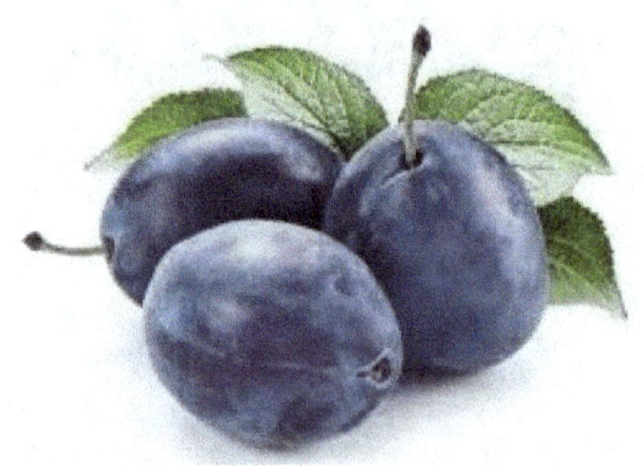

Radicchio also contains beta-carotene precursor of Vitamin A and, as well as figs, currants, blackberries and plums, potassium, which protects bone tissue and fights cardiovascular diseases and hypertension.

Eggplants, on the other hand, are rich in Magnesium, with the added advantage of having very few calories.

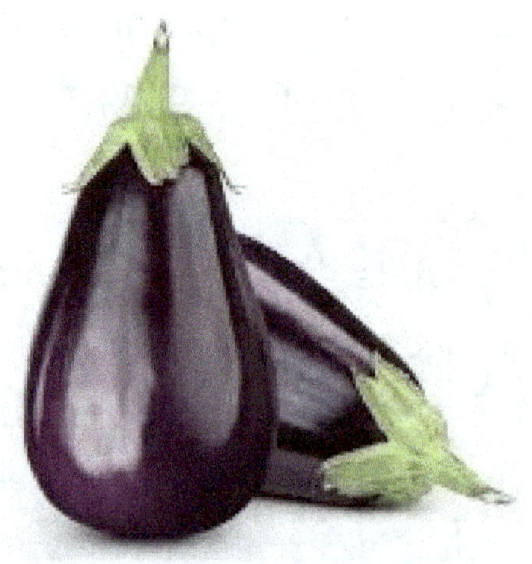

Finally, both fruit and vegetables of this color are rich in fiber and also in carotenoids, active against neuro-degenerative diseases and skin aging.

White.

Fruits and white vegetables strengthen the bone tissue and lungs.

Quercetin contained in these foods is a powerful antioxidant that defends 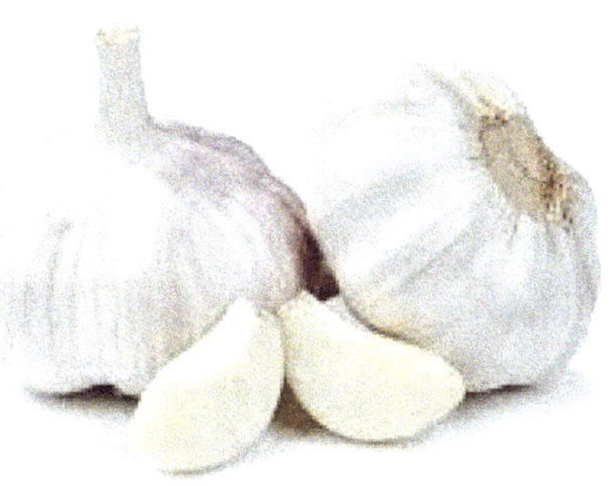 the body from the risk of cancer.

Rich in vitamins, fibers, potassium and other mineral salts, they also contain isothiocyanates, an excellent prevention tool against cellular aging.

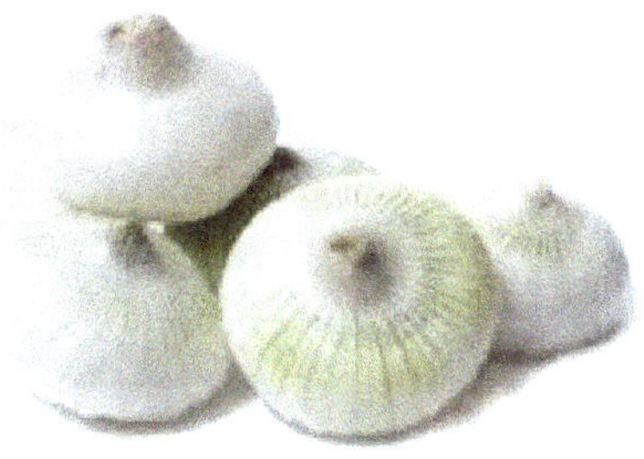 Garlic, onions and leeks also contain Allysulfide, which makes the blood more fluid and less prone to thrombus formation.

Selenium (found mainly in mushrooms) helps prevent hypertension.

And then, in addition to doing well, all these natural colors are a pleasure to see, at least this is my personal opinion.

to learn more: Antioxidants https://medlineplus.gov/antioxidants.html

SOME RECOMMENDED FOODS

Having clarified that the foods to be preferred for the Detox diet are foods of plant origin, specifically Fruits and Vegetables, below we talk about only some of them, but very important, describing in detail their characteristics.

Tomato, an elixir of youth.

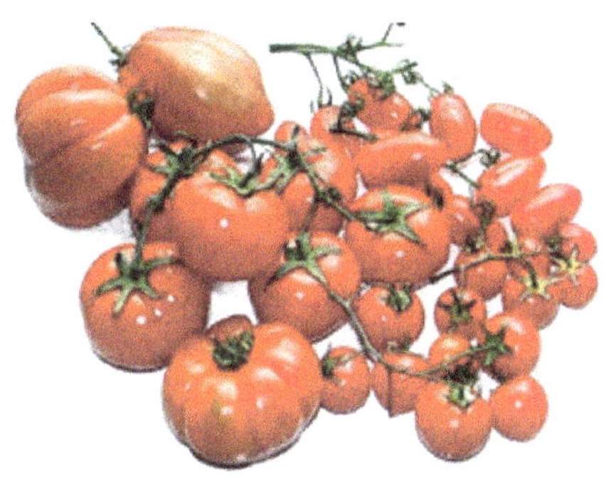

The tomato (Solanum lycopersicum) of the Solanaceae family (like potatoes, peppers and aubergines) is native to the area between the countries of Mexico and Peru today.

The Aztecs called it *"xitomatl"*, the term "tomatl" indicated various fruits similar to each other, usually juicy.

Tomato sauce was an integral part of Aztec cuisine.

According to some, the tomato had aphrodisiac properties, this is the reason why the French in ancient times called it "pomme d'amour", love apple.

Hernán Cortés was the tomato importer.

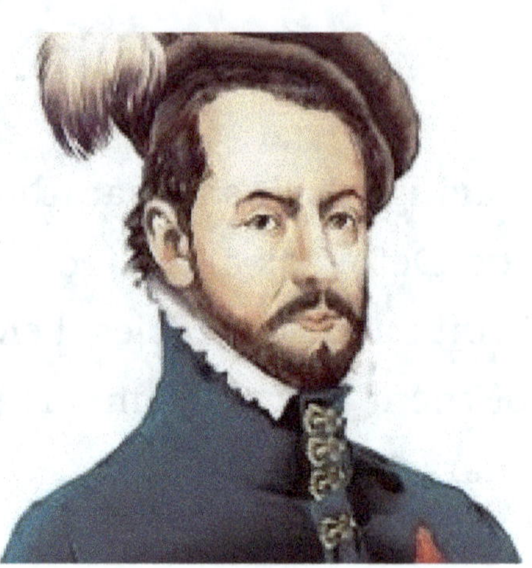

The tomato, in fact, arrived in Europe in 1540 when the Spaniard Hernán Cortés returned to his homeland and brought some specimens, but its cultivation and diffusion did not take place before the second half of the seventeenth century.

It arrived in Italy in 1596 but only later, finding favorable climatic conditions in the south of the country, did its color change from the original and characteristic gold color, which gave its name to the plant, to the current red, thanks to selections and subsequent grafts.

It is said that after its introduction in Europe Sir Walter Raleigh would have given this plant full of its fruits to Queen Elizabeth, baptizing it with the name of "apples of love".

For its goodness and beneficial properties it is one of the "best" vegetables, even if at first it was looked upon with a suspicious eye for its ideally dangerous fruits, the tomato, in the following years, was admired in botanical gardens as a plant typically exotic: currently, the tomato is appreciated for its malleability in the kitchen and for its properties in phytotherapy, and is a basis of the Mediterranean diet and, therefore, of the Mediterranean Zone.

Tomatoes are rich in water (94%), Carbohydrates represent almost the 3%, while the proteins are calculated around 1.2%, the fibers at 1% and, lastly, the fats represent only 0.2%.

For this reason, one hundred grams of fresh tomatoes provide only 17 Kcal.

From the point of view of the Zone Diet, **1 mini block** of Carbohydrates consists of 250g of ripe tomatoes or 300g of tomato puree, salad tomatoes, San Marzano tomatoes, tomato juice, peeled tomatoes, fruit and juice.

Tomatoes contain moderate quantities of vitamins: we recall **Vitamins of group B, ascorbic acid Vit. C, Vitamin D** and, above all, **Vitamin E**, which ensure the well-known **antioxidant** and vitaminizing properties of the tomato.

The mineral component is also abundant: Iron, Zinc, Selenium, Phosphorus and Calcium associated with citrates, tartrates and nitrates act in synergy ensuring remineralizing and anti-free radical properties which, together, favor cell repair and counteract aging in general. the whole organism - anti-aging action-.

They also have a moderate content of organic acids, such as malic, citric, succinic and glutenin, useful for promoting digestion.

From the point of view of health, the tomato is one of the most important vegetables.

It is a light, remineralizing, thirst-quenching food with high nutritional power and rich in flavor.

In fact, it provides few calories, with many minerals and trace elements and provides all the water-soluble vitamins.

Potassium, present in the dose of 298 mg per 100 g, helps the body, especially in summer, to regain water balance, to combat water retention and hypertension.

Also present are Calcium (9 mg), useful for the health of bones and teeth, and Phosphorus (25 mg) which helps us feel fit because it plays a fundamental role in many enzymatic processes and in muscle contraction.

What most distinguishes the tomato is a Carotenoid called Lycopene, the main pigment responsible for the red color of the tomato.

The tomato uses Lycopene to defend itself from damage

caused by the sun to its structure.

It should be noted that the tomato has the highest concentration of Lycopene in nature, i.e. from 30 to 400 mg / kg of fresh product.

Lycopene is also contained in smaller quantities in various fruits such as strawberry, papaya, melon, watermelon, grapes etc.

Lycopene has high antioxidant properties, even superior to those of Betacarotene.

In general, carotenoids are effective antioxidants, thanks to their effectiveness as a scavenger of free radicals. Among the Carotenoids, Lycopene seems to be the most efficient, thanks to the presence of two further double bonds with respect to the structure of the other Carotenoids.

From an increasing number of clinical studies, it is emerging that Lycopene brings multiple health benefits and, in particular, provides valid protection against various cancers.

The first researches have been stimulated by epidemiological studies that have highlighted a relationship between fruit and vegetable consumption in general and a decrease in the risk of certain types of cancer.

Several studies attribute to lycopene the ability to reduce

the risk of prostate cancer in humans, and experimental studies on mice suggest that it has the ability to suppress the growth of breast cancer cells.

The anti-cancer action of Lycopene has also been studied at the gastrointestinal, endometrial and skin levels.

Lycopene is also able to counteract cardiovascular diseases and delay the aging of the cells of our body.

Lycopene is able to counteract damage from sun exposure, improving skin density and protecting collagen fibers.

Lycopene is easily assimilated by the human body, largely in the fresh state and almost entirely when the tomato is subjected to the action of heat, in the presence of oil or other fats.

The tomato also contains organic acids, especially citric acid, responsible for the degree of acidity.

Thanks to this acidity, the tomato keeps quite a long time and the preserves can be treated only with heat without using any chemical preservative.

If fresh tomato is an exceptional Mediterranean food, perhaps less known are the concentrates, where the water is evaporated to increase the solid mass (or dry residue) and flavor.

While in the puree the dry residue is 6%, in the semi-concentrated it is higher than 12%, in the concentrate it is higher than 18%, in the double concentrated it is 28%. We also remind you that the heat favors the "extraction" of Lycopene and modifies its structure, making it more assimilable by the human body.

For this reason, fresh tomatoes contain only 3-5 mg of lycopene per 100 g, while in industrial products such as pulp, pureed and concentrated, the amount of lycopene is much higher.

This is the main reason why the use of tomato paste in the diet is also useful.

The concentrate can also become a simple and versatile secret to be used in the kitchen, to be used in vegetable soup, as in fish or meat, as well as to flavor a sandwich instead of using other sauces perhaps richer in fat and less flavor.

Since salt, i.e. sodium chloride, is usually already present in the products themselves, dishes based on tomato concentrate do not require adding more salt.

The result is lighter and healthier dishes.

Unlike the fresh fruit, which reaches its optimal level of flavor and usability only in the summer, the concentrate allows you to continue enjoying the virtues of this magnificent vegetable throughout the year, in an infinite variety of gluttons personalized menu for the Mediterranean Zone diet.

GARLIC

Certainly famous as a food, garlic (Allium sativum, Liliacee family) is also one of the most indispensable medicinal plants, being 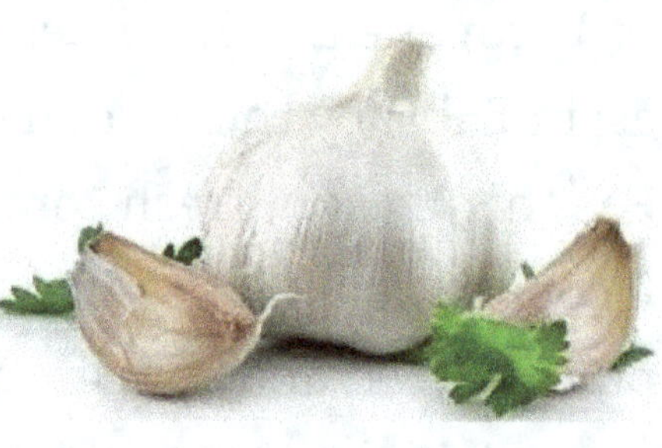 endowed with infinite health properties.

It is a herbaceous plant from 30 to 80 cm high, which in the wild is perennial, while if cultivated it propagates only vegetatively due to its sterility.

The garlic has a part that remains underground, consisting mainly of the bulb, covered with reddish casings and composed in turn of numerous smaller bulbs, the cloves, which provide the drug, or the part used in the phytotherapeutic field.

WHAT DOES THE SMELL COME FROM?

The typical smell of garlic is due to the sulfur compounds it contains, which form allicin in particular. Allicin is released when the allinase enzyme acts on alliin, a colorless and tasteless compound which is the main component of fresh drugs.

Garlic releases its characteristic smell every time it is crushed or cut as it happens during chewing, cutting, or squeezing.

The intact cloves, on the other hand, have no smell, because in intact cells alliin and other sulfoxides are contained in the cytoplasm, while its hydrolytic enzyme - allinase - is present only in the vacuole.

It is therefore necessary to destroy the cellular structure to release the aforementioned enzyme, which determines the hydrolysis of the sulfoxides, transforming them into disulfides and trisulphides.

VERY IMPORTANT ACTIVE INGREDIENTS

Allicin is a strong, remarkable antibiotic capable of inhibiting numerous types of bacteria, including those responsible for typhus, as was already noted in 1858 by Pasteur.

Garlic contains other antibacterial substances such as garlicina, and is rich in minerals and trace elements, such as magnesium, calcium, phosphorus, iodine and iron.

It also contains traces of zinc, manganese, selenium, vitamin C (only in fresh garlic), provitamin A, vitamins B1-B2-PP and also hormone-like substances and enzymes (lysozyme and peroxidase).

HEALING PROPERTIES

Among the many properties attributed to garlic is that of giving the skin a healthy appearance and promoting hair growth.

This effect is due to phytinic acid, which binds mineral substances and which can be transformed into inositol, a substance similar to vitamins capable of stimulating cell growth.

Garlic contains alkaloids with an action similar to that of insulin, lowering the level of blood sugar: this is why garlic is a valid support in therapies against diabetes and other diseases related to sugar metabolism.

It strengthens the immune system by acting as a powerful bactericide on the whole organism. It is a very powerful dewormer, a blood pressure regulator since it acts by causing vasodilation of the arterioles and capillaries, reduces the risk of sclerosis in the arteries, prevents the aggregation of platelets and the consequent formation of thrombus (therefore useful for vaccinated people). It also has the ability to regulate the level of cholesterol and triglycerides in the blood.

ANTIBIOTIC FUNCTION

Fundamental is its characteristic antibiotic function, having bacteriostatic and bactericidal action both against Gram + and Gram - bacteria.

In fact, garlic is an important antibiotic that can be used when the intestinal bacterial flora has been altered by previous treatments.

Given that, unlike synthetic antibiotics, while garlic attacks pathogenic bacteria but does not damage the saprophytic bacterial flora, favoring their restoration instead.

Garlic is an excellent remedy for bloating and abdominal cramps, and is also very useful in case of acute and chronic diarrhea or mucus-bloody stools (dysentery).

Studies show its activity against Helicobacter pylori, the bacterium partly responsible for gastric ulcer and also for the development of stomach tumors.

PROTECTS FROM HEAVY METALS.

Garlic has the ability to protect against heavy metals, very dangerous substances that enter the body through polluted air and contaminated food.

The most exposed organs are the lungs, kidneys, liver and nervous system, with effects that can give immediate symptoms but also pathological manifestations after years.

Garlic acts as a chelator, ie the sulfur compounds present in its molecules bind stably to the molecules of mercury, lead and cadmium present in the body, allowing their elimination easily.

You can learn more here

PINE NUTS

They are the edible seeds of some species of pine, in particular the pine Pinus pinea.

They are therefore contained in the pine cone, or rather, in the strobilus, a "pseudo-fruit" aimed at protecting and propagating the small seeds of the plant in the environment.

NUTRITIONAL CHARACTERISTICS

Like other oil seeds, pine nuts are also extremely energetic, primarily for lipids (50% of the weight of a dry pine nut).

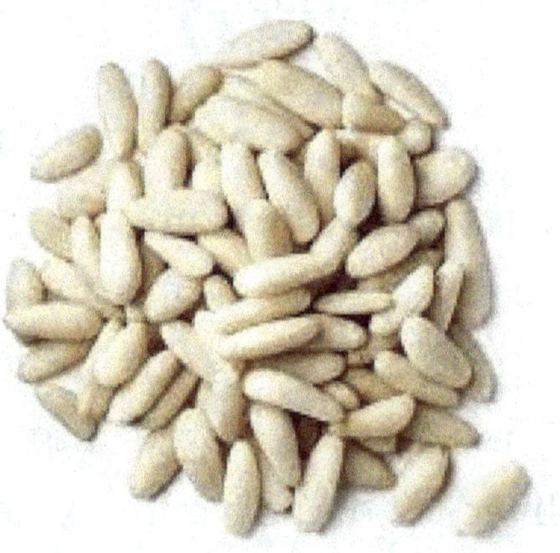

Completely cholesterol-free, they instead contain high amounts of triglycerides, consisting of mainly unsaturated and therefore good fatty acids, due to the EXCELLENT supply of linoleic acid (an essential polyunsaturated with a cholesterol-lowering function).

The pine nuts also have a good protein content (30%

of the weight), with a content of amino acids which determines a fairly good biological value; the main amino acids are: glutamic acid, arginine and aspartic acid, while the limiting amino acid is lysine.

Remember that in the human body, arginine is considered the main precursor of nitric oxide, a molecule capable of optimizing the physiological dilation of blood vessels.

They are also a great source of dietary fiber (4.5% by weight).

The amount of carbohydrates, on the other hand, does not greatly affect the total energy intake.

MINERAL SALTS AND VITAMINS

Pine nuts are rich in iron and phosphorus but also interesting for manganese, potassium, zinc and copper.

As for vitamins, the tocopherols (**vitamin E**) are especially important in pine nuts, with valuable antioxidant characteristics.

The levels of thiamine (**vit. B1**), riboflavin (**vit. B2**) and niacin (**vit. PP**) are also interesting.

Excellent for those who play sports, they are to be consumed carefully by overweight subjects, since 100g of dry seeds provide about 600Kcal.

UTILITIES

They are useful for improving the lipid profile of hypercholesterolemia patients and, given the considerable presence of arginine, they can be useful against hypertension.

They are indicated in growth, in pregnancy (if you are not allergic) and in conditions characterized by asthenia since some hypothesize that pine nuts are energizing regardless of calorie intake).

They are not particularly suitable for breastfeeding because they are responsible for a slight taste alteration of the milk. Pine nuts are an excellent alternative to other types of dried fruit.

The average portion of pine nuts corresponds to about 1 tablespoon per day, equal to approximately 60kcal.

OREGANO

Oregano, seasoning and medicine. Spices and herbs are often overlooked substances in our diet, although they have been shown to contain even greater beneficial amounts of anti-aging substances than other plant foods.

We use few of them and in our kitchen almost exclusively the flavors of parsley, celery, sage and rosemary have space.

Thyme, oregano, savory, coriander, cumin, chives, mint, dill, bay leaf (just to name a few) are spices that we should know and use more.

In general they have great anti-defective power and are therefore to be used particularly in winter to fight infectious diseases, but also energetic and anti-aging, thanks to their unparalleled antioxidant properties.

These are valuable activities for the nerve cells whose very intense activity produces many free radicals that need to be blocked by large quantities of antioxidants.

They are all important to our health and we should get used to using them more often and in greater numbers.

Here we delve into oregano. Oregano (Origanum vulgare) is a perennial shrub widely used in Mediterranean cuisine.

It belongs to the genus Origanum, which groups about fifty herbaceous, evergreen or semi-permanent leaf species that are part of the Lamiaceae family together with marjoram and mint.

It grows spontaneously in sunny and arid places up to 2,000 meters above sea level.

This is why its name means "joy of the mountain" (from the Greek "oros" meaning mountain and "ganos" which means splendor, delight).

It is also called acciughero or anchovy herb because it

is used to flavor anchovy paste and also bastard mint because the bushes smell slightly of mint. it is a typically Mediterranean spice, although examples are found in Siberia and in the Himalayan regions.

Good quality oregano has an intense aroma.

The climate, the season and the soil influence the composition and concentration of the essential oils present in the plant.

Varieties that grow in cold climates are often lacking in taste.

The branches can be dried and stored away from air and light.

Dried oregano has a more intense flavor than fresh.

With drying, contrary to what happens to parsley or basil, the aroma of oregano is preserved, becoming stronger and more concentrated.

Thanks to the destruction of plant tissues, in fact, essential oils are more available, spreading more easily in food.

Very fragrant is the southern oregano (Origanum heracleoticum), widespread in southern Italy and the islands, a fundamental ingredient of pizza and many other Mediterranean dishes (for the recipe for PIZZA in the Zone click here).

Appreciated since ancient times for its beneficial

properties, **Oregano** is widely used for both food and therapeutic purposes.

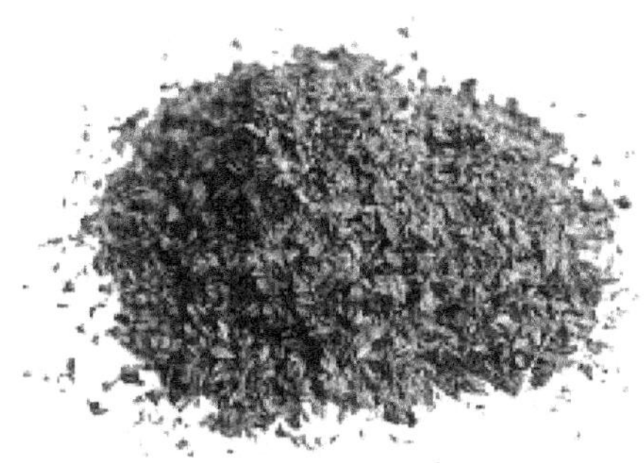

Due to its characteristics, **Oregano** is considered a plant that gives comfort, relief and health. In ancient times, thanks to its penetrating scent, it was used as a disinfectant for environments during epidemics.

It is currently used in aromatherapy, cosmetics and pharmacology.

Thanks to the activity of the essential oils contained in it, thymol and carvacrol, oregano has calming properties, helps difficult digestion, blocks nervous nausea, promotes sleep and is a good diuretic.

In medicine, moreover, it is used to thin bronchial secretions, as an antiseptic of the respiratory tract and as a sedative, antitoxic, antiviral, bactericide and febrifuge. Given its antibacterial properties, it can be useful in the treatment of acne and candida infections. Oregano is also a good repellent for ants: just sprinkle it in frequented places and remember to replace it often.

In addition to ants, it is unwelcome to numerous other parasites so it is useful to grow it close to other plants that protects it from a whole series of infections.

If used pure on the skin it can cause irritation but the flowers, collected in a bunch and slightly heated, are also an excellent remedy against a stiff neck.

Oregano is a very powerful antioxidant, apparently more powerful than garlic and blueberry. Oregano contains an anti-inflammatory substance, **beta-caryophilene**.

The substance has effects on inflammation, pain, atherosclerosis and osteoporosis.

It is present not only in oregano but also in other aromatic plants such as basil and rosemary and in some spices including cinnamon and black pepper.

Beta-caryophyllene acts on the receptive structures of cell membranes, the so-called CB2 receptors, modifying the behavior of the cells.

It works in the same way as the Endocannabinoids produced by the same cells in our body.

When inflammation breaks out, endocannabinoids ensure that the immune system does not have an "excessive" reaction, that is, aggravating the inflammatory process.

Unlike other substances such as Cannabis and Opioids, which also bind to CB2 receptors, the beta-caryophyllene of oregano has no intoxicating effect.

Hence the pharmacological interest in this substance,

which according to many researchers could form the basis for the development of new drugs to control some chronic inflammatory diseases, starting with Crohn's disease, which mainly affects the intestine.

Avoid using Oregano in case of gastritis, peptic ulcer, dermatitis or ascertained hypersensitivity to one or more components.

The use of oregano is not even considered in the calculation of the blocks for the Zone diet.

Mackerel

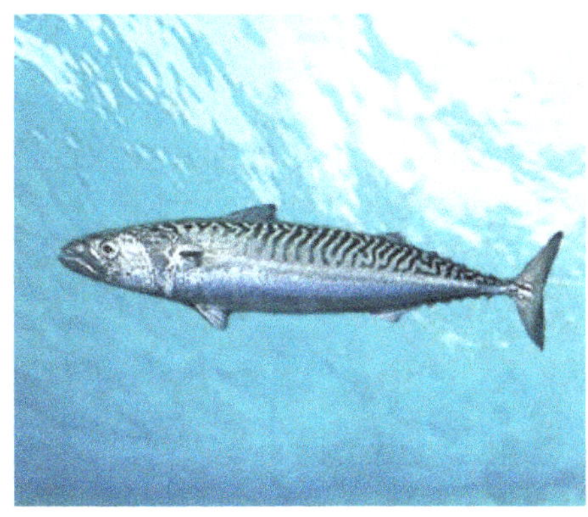

Mackerel (Scomber scombrus), is a sea fish belonging to the Scombridae family.

They are typical representatives of the blue fish.

Mackerel is about 25-50 cm long with a fusiform body and pointed head.

Being a voracious predator, the mackerel has a wide mouth with jaws equipped with small sharp teeth.

Mackerel live in flocks throughout the Mediterranean, the North Sea and the North Atlantic. From a nutritional point of view it is a food that we can define as exceptional since, like all other species belonging to blue fish, mackerel are also particularly rich in polyunsaturated fatty acids. In addition to protecting against cardiovascular diseases, this abundant presence of "good" fats gives the meat a distinctive, decisive and tasty flavor.

It is also rich in easily digestible proteins and has a modest caloric intake.

1 block of Mackerel protein consists of 40g

It is sold fresh, frozen or processed and canned.

Being particularly widespread in our seas, it has a low price.

Mackerel is one of the most used and appreciated fish of the Mediterranean diet and is recommended by Nutritionists and the Mediterranean Zone Diet for its contribution in Omega-3 fats, particularly suitable for those suffering from hypercholesterolemia.

In 100g of Mackerel there are:

C20: 5 W3 (Eicosapentaenoic - EPA) 0.73 g

C22: 6 W3 (Docosahexaenoic - DHA) 1.26 g

Tot EPA + DHA per 100g = 1.99g per meal of 3 blocks 2.4g

of EPA + DHA are ingested while for 4 blocks 3.2 g of EPA + DHA are ingested.

The daily requirement of EPA + DHA is generally considerate, according to different situations, between 0.5 to 2.5g / day.

Let's not forget that Omega-3s, not very common in nature, are also found in Mediterranean plant foods such as almonds.

A tasty and quick way to eat fish and Omega 3 (and also cheap). 3 or 4 blocks Chop, fine or thick according to taste, with carrot 120g 1C + onion 80g 1/2 C + 1 stalk of celery and 2 cloves of garlic not counted, pepper + a little salt. grease the pan with 1 tablespoon of 1G oil.

When the onion is golden, add 150g of tomato sauce 1 / 2C and sprinkle with oregano.

As soon as everything is blended, add 120g 3P or 160g 4P of cleaned fresh mackerel fillets. Cook for 5 minutes or so.

These are 3 blocks of protein with about 6 blocks of G or 4 blocks of P with close to 7 blocks of G, but we can stay with that as they are mostly good or very good fats.

The blocks of C are still 2 and therefore we will have either 1 or 2 C blocks left over, depending on whether we make a meal of 3 or 4 blocks. If we add vegetables such as radicchio or salad which are worth 0 C, we are left with 115/230g of oranges or 130/260 of apricots.

For other fruit, consult the tables that can be downloaded by those who took the test (even without purchasing our Personalized Diet).

THE ZONE AT A GLANCE

At this point, having clarified the characteristics of the Detox diet, it will be sufficient to use these detoxifying foods using the parameters of the Zone.

What are the important points for a correct diet in the area?

Many mistakenly believe that the Zone diet is complicated, but by reading the various points below, you realize that it is just a matter of using common sense, associated with simple notions. On this page I clearly explain what you need to know.

Balance Carbohydrates-Proteins-Fat.

A dose of Carbohydrates, one of Proteins and one of Fats must never be missing.

An adequate amount of protein, low in saturated fat, is also essential, such as to provide 30% total calories and finally a moderate amount of fat, preferably monounsaturated, such as to provide 30% of total calories.

Give preference to healthier foods.

It is better to use foods rich in nutrients such as vitamins, mineral salts, fiber, etc. and therefore with "healthy" characteristics and defined for this favorable, compared to those poor in nutrients and containing substances harmful to the body (saturated fats-trans-arachidonic acid, etc.) defined as **unfavorable** for this.

In practice this means eating more fruits and vegetables (favorable carbohydrates) more fish, white meats and low-fat dairy products (favorable proteins), and using olive oil as a condiment, or as a snack almonds, pistachios, cashews (all sources of fat. good).

In this, the classic zone also coincides perfectly with the Detox.

Distribute the food throughout the day.

This will allow you to maintain hormonal balance throughout the day.

The consequence will be never to be hungry but to lose weight anyway if and when necessary. Never go fasting.

It is important never to fast for more than 5 hours, except when sleeping.

Always remember that each meal provides nutrients and regulates our hormonal system for about 4-6 hours while each snack for about 2-3 hours.

Water is not only a fundamental constituent of our body but, more specifically, it is also essential if you want to lose weight.

If, of course, a lot of fruit and vegetables are consumed, the water to drink is necessarily less.

The Zone.

It is not necessary to be obsessively rigid in following these indications since the Mediterranean Zone diet is an extremely flexible food strategy.

Just know that it will be more effective the more it is followed.

The Zone, therefore, is not the usual diet that imposes a rigid and restrictive dietary protocol to be followed in a rigorous and passive way.

These diets - low-calorie, high-protein - often lead to discomfort and frustration and for this reason they easily end up being abandoned.

A **Zone** diet allows you to learn the correct way to eat from a hormonal and genetic point of view.

Once we understand the fundamental concepts based on solid and proven scientific bases, it will be possible to manage our diet for life, choosing from a large number of foods.

It will thus be possible to become directly responsible for your own health and well-being.

Each meal and / or snack becomes a new opportunity to positively or negatively affect one's hormones, thus becoming directly responsible for one's health and well-being.

This also means that if during a dinner or lunch you happen to "overdo it" it will not be necessary to be overwhelmed by feelings of guilt but it will be sufficient for the next meal to be in the Zone to restore hormonal balance.

It will thus be possible to return to the Zone, that is, in that state of maximum harmony and hormonal balance which translates into greater *Health and Energy* and in a *Weight Loss* if necessary.

When starting a new type of correct nutrition like the Zone, we have to take into account many things.

In particular, there are factors that should not be underestimated to do the right thing.

On this page I outline the fundamental factors we need to take into account.

Specifically, I deal with the following aspects: A psychobiological phenomenon.

There are many factors to keep in mind when setting one's diet correctly, considering that, as mentioned elsewhere, nutrition does not only serve to provide the essential energy we use to live, but it is actually a complex psychobiological phenomenon, rich in multiple physical and psychological implications.

Satisfy the taste.

The first characteristic that any diet (meaning this term in its original sense of the way you eat) must have, is to satisfy the *"sense of taste"* of the person concerned, thus gratifying his palate.

With this we do not mean that it is appropriate to eat only the foods we have a sweet tooth, but it is equally true that diets made only of "right" but unwelcome foods, not only end up making life less beautiful, but simply after some time they come abandoned.

Virtually all the foods available to us and to our greater or lesser liking can and must find a place in our diet. It is about learning to balance the various nutrients in order to satisfy our tastes and at the same time provide the body with everything it needs.

Physical activity is essential.

We must never forget, then, that we belong to the Animal Kingdom and that, therefore, the necessary complement to nutrition is physical activity, without which multiple physiological functions, including digestive processes, end up worsening.

It is precisely physical activity, in fact, that will determine a substantial portion of our energy needs, consequently determining how much we can eat.

Distribute meals throughout the day.

It is also important how we eat, or how the meals are distributed throughout the day.

In fact, it is not the same thing to ingest, for example, 2000 K.cal all together, in a single meal, or to take the same amount of food in several meals throughout the day.

The possibility of gaining weight will be greater in the first case than in the second, this is because every time we eat, part of the energy taken is "spent" to activate the digestive processes. it is therefore strongly recommended to distribute the food several times.

Normally it is recommended to have 5 meals a day, obviously not all the same.

Use the "*good*" fats.

A myth to dispel is that all fats are bad for you.

In reality, animal fats are the ones that are risky to health, while vegetable fats, or oils and in particular olive oil, in addition to performing fundamental functions, help keep our arteries clean.

A daily pattern.

A daily scheme of proper nutrition in the Zone could therefore be the following:

- Breakfast (absolutely essential in the morning, upon awakening).

- Second breakfast in the middle of the morning, so as not to be too hungry for lunch.

- Lunch (with a large dose of vegetables in addition to proteins).

- Mid-afternoon snack, so as not to be too hungry for dinner.

- Dinner (with a large dose of vegetables in addition to proteins).

- ELIMINATE OUT OF MEAL!

The energy requirement.
The growth of our body depends on proper nutrition and consequently the food intake must be adequate to the needs, both from an energy point of view, i.e. calories, and from a point of view of the percentage composition of the various substances.
During the first 20 years of life we need 2,500 kg of carbohydrates (sugars and carbohydrates are

synonymous), 300 kg of proteins, 625 kg of lipids (i.e. fats), 2,500,000 liters of oxygen and 33,000 liters of water, as well as vitamins and minerals.

Water is essential.

The composition of the human body. Since an adult eliminates about 2.5 liters of water a day in urine, sweat, feces and water vapor emitted by breathing, it is evident how these losses must be compensated for by food: even if most foods contains a 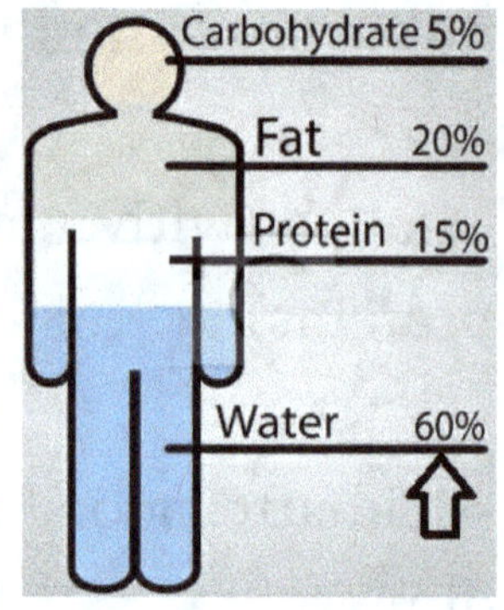

good amount of water such as fruit and vegetables, which contain 90%, meat 70%, bread 35%, you need to drink at least one and a half liters a day.

Water is necessary so as not to burden the work of the kidneys, to hydrate the tissues and to eliminate toxins.

Importance of Proteins.

As for the protein intake, necessary for the construction of the proteins of which the tissues of the human body are made, remember that only proteins contain nitrogen atoms, necessary to synthesize the proteins themselves.

To get an idea of the percentage of proteins contained in some foods, remember that about 50 grams of them are contained in 250 grams of meat, in 5 eggs, in about 1 and a half liters of milk, 200 grams of cheese or dried legumes.

However, not all proteins are similar, since the percentage of amino acids that compose them varies: there are those of animal origin and those of vegetable origin (for example those of soy). And since the proteins contained in the different foods are different from each other, it is necessary to mix meat or fish, milk, cheese, legumes, to obtain the right balance. If you are **Vegan**, you will need to make the correct dosage of vegetable proteins for a correct diet in the area.

MY ENGLISH BOOKS ON AMAZON

our Zone diet from a Mediterranean point of view!

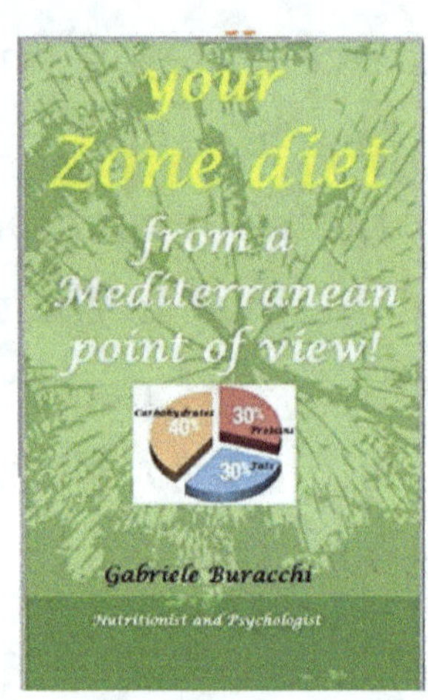

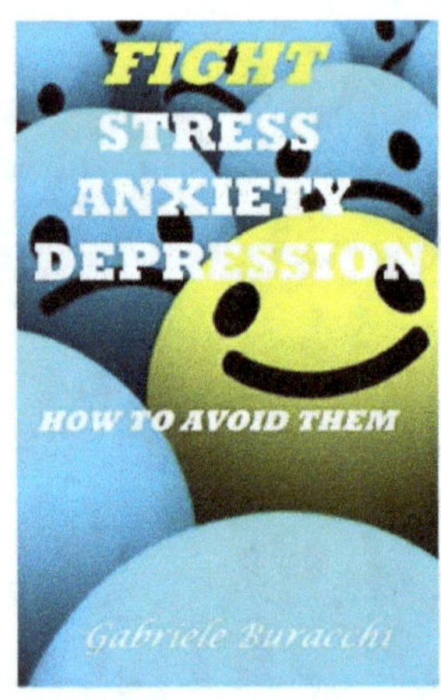

FIGHT STRESS, ANXIETY, DEPRESSION: what are they, how to recognize them, how to avoid them

Prostate. Instructions for Use !: What are the problems of the Prostate? Prevent and treat them with nutrition, natural products and the

right physical activity

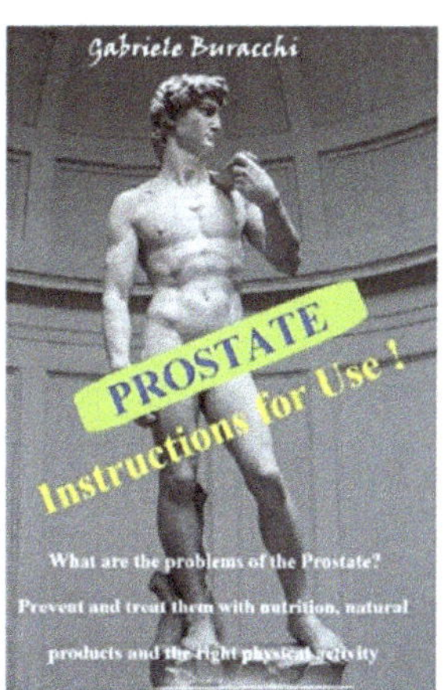

YOU CAN WRITE ME IN ENGLISH,FRENCH, SPANISH, ITALIAN at

gab.bur@yandex.com

my italian website

www.dietazonaonline.com